THE CAUSES AND TREATMENT OF WOMEN'S AILMENTS

The ailments which cause suffering and inconvenience to so many modern women are always preventable – and nearly always curable when they are properly understood. The Nature Cure system of treatment described in this book can be self-applied at home because it dispenses with dangerous drugs and surgery.

# The Causes and Treatment of Women's Ailments

Isa Anderson Kelso N.D., M.B.N.O.A.

THORSONS PUBLISHERS LIMITED
Wellingborough, Northamptonshire

First published 1958
Second Impression 1964
Third Impression 1969
Second Edition, revised and reset, 1973
Second Impression 1976
Third Impression 1978
Fourth Impression 1981
Fifth Impression 1983





ISBN 0 7225 0219 2

Printed and bound in Great Britain

# Contents

# 1.
# General Principles

THIS BOOK HAS been written to give women some enlightenment about the many common yet nearly always preventable ailments of their sex. For years women had accepted poor health as part of their lot because they were supposed to be the weaker sex. Happily this outlook has now completely changed. Women have proved in innumerable ways that they compare very favourably in physical fitness with men, and modern investigations have established that the majority of women's ailments need never occur.

Most people do not realize that disease occurring in adults usually originates in infancy. Unfortunately all children are not born healthy, which means that we do not all have an equal chance to enjoy good health. It will easily be understood that it is much more difficult to cure an unhealthy child or grown-up who has had the misfortune to be born into this world in a weakened state than a person who has acquired ill-health in infancy.

In a way it is fortunate, therefore, that most of us do acquire our disabilities in the first few years of our lives, due mainly to wrong feeding, because cure then becomes much easier. Most of these troubles arise because the majority of mothers do not understand what the upsets of infancy really signify. Wrong treatment then undoubtedly leads to much of the adult illness.

It is this lack of knowledge of the ability of the body to effect its own healing, which allows a mother to administer the well-known medicinal aids such as soothing powders, purgatives and mild sedatives. It is all too common to find aspirin given even to an infant to ease restlessness which may be coming merely from a very over-loaded stomach.

The majority of children appear slightly better after such treatment so the mother accepts this as a cure and unfortunately decides to apply the same method when they again become ill. Actually what has really happened is that nature, in her first attempt to cleanse, has been thwarted and has stopped her efforts momentarily because, not only has she the original impurity to cleanse, but she has now to deal with the additional debris resulting from the drug.

The initial efforts to clean the system usually manifest themselves in the form of colds, fevers, skin eruptions, vomiting and diarrhoea. When these are checked and the clogging material forced back into the child's system, then the first foundations of disease impurity are laid.

Nature Cure, on which this book is based, teaches that as children grow, they tend to correct inherited weaknesses and that they do so by elimination. The extent of this elimination is measured by the inherent vitality of the body and is present in every child at birth, to a greater or less degree, according to the health of the child. It shows in the cleansings of the child's system which manifest themselves in the acute illnesses already mentioned. If these upsets were treated by natural methods, results would be good and a much larger percentage of adolescents and grown-ups would be enjoying real health.

Our bodies constantly accumulate debris from the breaking up and renewing of our tissue cells. Nature has created the means to rid our bodies of this by an eliminative process, functioning through main channels, namely, the kidneys, bowel, lungs and skin. These organs can become so clogged and overworked that they are quite unfit to perform in a normal manner, with the result that incomplete elimination allows impurities to pile up within the body.

Not every women is endowed with perfect health, but most women's troubles are the result of suppressive treatment in early life and could be prevented by applying a little knowledge and common sense. Where layer upon layer of disease impurity has collected over a period of years by constant suppression of acute illnesses, the inherent vitality of the body becomes low and complete cure may be impossible. Even at this stage, however, a great deal of help can be obtained from natural methods of healing.

Nature Cure methods allow the body to do its own cleansing. It does so by increasing the eliminative powers by diet, exercise and water treatments, until they gradually remove accumulated impurity. The methods in this book are simple and can be applied at home. If, however, a trouble has progressed until it is really serious it is wiser to consult a trained Nature Cure practitioner, because other methods not suitable for home treatment may be required. Psychological upsets may be the cause or displacement of any one or more of the bony structures of the body which may have occurred. The latter must be corrected by manipulation because they usually result from accidents, falls or severe blows. Displacement can, however, affect one or more of the vital organs and so cause loss of rhythm in an organ far removed from the source of the trouble. In such cases it is advisable to consult a naturopath for examination and manipulative treatment.

For those who are able to treat their ailments at home I would emphasize the fact that a slow gradual improvement is to be desired, rather than a quick result. Often the upset has taken years to manifest itself and days or a few weeks will not correct the damage. The diet and regime advised here will, however, give lasting results provided they are strictly observed. Nature will not be hurried, and by obeying her laws perfect health, beyond the dreams of the sufferer, can often be attained.

# 2.
# Feeding for Health

IN NATURAL HEALING, the taking of a balanced dietary is the basic part of the treatment. There are few people with any experience of the subject who will deny that our health depends largely upon what we eat, and to give some idea of the value of food is advisable as many people constantly eat wrongly balanced meals.

During the last quarter of a century plain wholesome foods have almost completely disappeared and have been replaced by artificial, processed, adulterated and deficient foods, lacking in mineral salts and natural vitamins so necessary to the maintaining of good health. The taking of these devitalized foods results in the natural mineral salts of the body being burned up and never replenished, and this factor alone can be the underlying cause of certain ailments especially found in women.

Nature Cure diets are arranged slightly differently for each complaint, but I would like every diet to be built on the approximate following percentages.

50 per cent Vegetables and fruit.
25 per cent Protein and fat foods.
25 per cent Starchy and sugar foods.

The meaning of these terms will be explained later in this chapter.

Such an ideal arrangement may not always be possible or suitable, but this is the near-perfect diet and eating in something likes these proportions would definitely result in a great improvement in health.

**Vegetables and Fruits**

Eating vegetables in quantity each day is essential in

order to supply certain mineral salts required for body chemistry. It is a regrettable fact that almost every adult is suffering from a lack of some of these salts.

The percentage of mineral salts and vitamins is much higher when the vegetables are obtained fresh and are grown on compost-manured ground. Not every one possesses a garden and can grow vegetables in this way, but more and more commercial growers are becoming aware that artificially manured vegetables are lacking in balance and many are now turning to natural methods of growing. The health of the people will gradually benefit by this. Shortage of mineral salts intake is always serious and vegetables must be taken twice daily, preferably one raw meal and the other cooked. The green vegetables are the most valuable and must be eaten every day.

Fruits are also a great aid to balanced dieting. They are divided into two main classes, fresh and dried. The first class consists of apples, oranges, grapefruit, pears, grapes, lemons, plums, and when digestion is normal and the stomach healthy, their reaction is alkaline, although some are acid to taste. They are not advisable, however, in certain ailments at the beginning of treatment and special notes will be found about them in the treatment of these complaints. Dried fruits, such as prunes, figs, raisins, apricots, are acid in reaction unless they are soaked overnight and then simmered, when they are invaluable as bowel cleansers.

Fruit is used principally for its cleansing action and to introduce mineral salts and vitamins into the body. It corrects any acidity of the blood and a daily intake of fresh and dried fruit is necessary for the prevention of serious illness based on vitamin shortage.

## Proteins

These foods build and repair tissues which are continually wearing and require renewing. It is in youth that this type of food is most vital. The average adult eats far too many proteins but as we grow older our growth and development are slowed and therefore there is not the same demand for tissue replacement. In fact there are certain states of ill-health where proteins, except in very small quantities, can be highly injurious. These points will be explained when these particular ailments are being dealt with later in this book.

The principal protein foods are meat, fish, fowl, cheese, peas, brans, lentils, nuts and milk. There is no actual necessity to take flesh protein, because it does not supply any greater food value than the others and it places more strain on the eliminating organs. One protein daily is sufficient, and to ensure balance and aid digestion, vegetables and fruit should be taken with the protein meal.

### Fats

Only a small amount of fat is required for health and this should be chosen from butter, nut butter, inorganic nut oil and olive oil.

### Sugars and Starches

Heat and energy are supplied from these foods and the best sugars are Barbados sugar, honey, molasses, dates and raisins. Most people eat too many sugary foods and these can cause a great deal of digestive upset.

The starches are all cereals and certain vegetables such as potatoes. They are also required to furnish heat and energy on digestion and are frequently overeaten, causing clogging of the tissues and increasing the formation of catarrh. It is always advisable to take some form of raw vegetable with the starchy meal.

In Nature Cure diets, certain foods are not advised as they come within the category of deficient foods. These are all white flour products, white sugar, manufactured sugar, condiments, preserves, pastries, refined cereals, milk puddings, fried and greasy foods and tinned foods.

Most people also drink too much fluid. Many of these fluids, such as tea, coffee, aerated waters and all alcoholic drinks, are extremely injurious. The best fluids are water, vegetable and fruit juices, vegetable soup (made without meat), butter-milk, koumiss and yogurt. Even these should be taken in moderation except where advised, especially by those who are overweight.

# 3. Suggested General Diet

BREAKFAST

Fresh acid fruit such as apples, oranges, pears, grapes and grapefruit, in any quantity and mixture.

One glass of cold milk. (Unpasteurized.)

This mixture is building yet cleansing and the milk protein combines excellently with the fresh acid fruit.

MID-MORNING

Fresh fruit only. Water to drink when thirsty.

LUNCH

Protein such as egg dish or cheese dish or raw grated cheese, or peas, beans or lentils.

Steamed or casseroled vegetables. (Particularly the green variety.)

Dessert: Fresh acid fruit.

This is an excellent way to arrange the protein part of the meal, and it ensures good assimiliation because it makes the protein more easily digested, and prevents overeating when the starchy potatoes are not included.

EVENING MEAL

Steamed vegetables or raw vegetable salad should always be included in this meal and steamed or baked potatoes may be added in the form of wholemeal bread or toast, or any crisp bread.

Butter, dates, figs, raisins or honey. Olive oil and lemon juice as salad dressing.

The dried fruits may be added to the salad if preferred. No proteins are advised with the starchy meal.

SUPPER

Fresh fruit only.

FLUIDS: Any of the fluids already suggested may be taken in small quantities and always between meals.

This is a general guide to the form of balanced dieting because we believe that the kitchen is where the main causes of ill-health originate. Faulty nutrition is the start of the majority of the ailments.

# 4.
# Water Treatments

---

WATER IS LARGELY used in Nature Cure to increase the flow of the blood and lymphatic circulations, because there is often a fundamental sluggishness of circulation as an underlying factor in all ailments. Without going into greater detail it will be readily understood that hot applications dilate the blood vessels and thereby slow the circulation and very often relieve pain. On the other hand, when cold water is applied there is no great relief of pain (although it does occur in certain cases such as neuritis) but the circulation is very much speeded up in the reaction.

## Alternate Hot and Cold Applications

These are widely used and are best applied by preparing two packs of linen or cotton material of a thickness which will retain a considerable amount of fluid. The pack is first soaked in hot water, wrung out and applied to the part and retained there for two minutes. It is then removed and immediately followed by a cold pack which is kept on for one minute. The hot application is then applied again for two minutes followed by the cold for another minute, and so on for ten or fifteen minutes, always finishing with the cold pack.

Alternate hot and cold applications are safe and can be used over any inflamed part without the slightest degree of danger. This is most important, because the application of heat itself is often attended with considerable risk as if there is inflammation below the part which is painful, the heat may 'draw' it and cause rupture. This would be a dangerous reaction in the case of appendicitis, gastric ulceration or in ear troubles and therefore the hot application alone should never be used except under the direction of a Nature Cure practitioner.

## The Cold Compress

In the practice of Nature Cure, the cold compress is used as a means of stimulating the circulation of any part of the body. Its reaction increases the drainage of the part and promotes healing. There are certain factors, however, about compressing which must be emphasized, otherwise more harm than good will result. The following rules should be carefully studied:

(1) Never apply a compress when you are feeling tired.

(2) Never apply a compress immediately before or during the menstrual period. Make sure that the compress heats up within minutes of application or it may do harm.

(3) Make sure that the compress heats up within minutes of application or it may do harm.

(4) Remove a cold damp compress immediately to avoid chilling.

(5) Wash the linen of the compress after each application. In many cases a considerable amount of poisonous debris is drawn through the skin by the compress and this must be removed, otherwise it may be re-absorbed.

(6) Never apply a local compress without having one on the waist. If a local compress is used when the system is very toxic, then there is a tendency to bring more impurities to the part and this may cause more trouble.

**The Waist Compress**

Here is a description of how the waist compress is applied. Take a piece of linen, cotton or cheese cloth, about six to ten inches broad and long enough to go round the waist. The compress may be fastened with safety pins, but a much better method is to provide the linen with tapes. Soak the linen in cold water, wring it out and place firmly, but not too tightly, around the waist. Fix with the tapes or safety pins, then cover it with two or three layers of warm material such as flannel or wool. This should overlap the wet compress in every direction. Usually the compress is applied before retiring, but of course, it can be used at any time in feverish conditions. It should heat up within a few minutes of application. This can be ascertained by inserting the fingers between the skin and the compress when a moist heat will be felt. If this heat is not present within fifteen minutes, remove the compress and give the skin a brisk rub with a rough towel, continuing until a red flush is seen. This will prevent any chilling of the affected part.

It will often be found that the back of the body does not react as vigorously as the front. If this occurs, increase the amount of covering over the back of the compress or place a hot water bag near the part. In some cases experience proves that the back will not heat up and the compress is then reduced or cut short and this part is left uncovered by the wet linen. Although this procedure is allowed it greatly reduces the efficiency of the compress and as the vitality of the body rises, then the size of the compress should be increased. Sometimes the compress heats up but before it becomes dry, a feeling of chill arises and the chest appears damp. Remove it immediately and give the skin a brisk towelling. After the compress has been removed the part of the skin covered by it should be thoroughly washed with warm soapy water and then cold water. If any form of skin outbreak appears, stop the application for the time being and wash the parts thoroughly and frequently with warm soapy water. This is a sign that the compress is drawing a great deal of impurity through the skin and when this skin outbreak disappears, the compress can be used normally.

**The Sitz Bath**

This is an old-fashioned, but still highly beneficial method of using water as a healing agent. Ideally it should be practised in a special form of hip bath designed for the purpose, but as these are not readily obtainable in this country the ordinary bath is most frequently used. Fill the bath with water, up to say twelve inches, then immerse the hips and abdomen but attempt to keep the feet, legs and the rest of the body clear of the water. A stool placed in the bath will make it easier to keep the legs up and the arms will support the rest of the body. If alternate hot and cold Sitz baths are advised, the cold one should be provided by a large basin placed beside the bath.

Alternate hot and cold Sitz baths are given to retone the organs of the lower abdomen and are of very great value in ailments of the reproductive organs, in bladder conditions, and where there is abdominal prolapse. They remove inflammation and bring back muscular tone into the affected parts. If this form of bathing was practised more regularly, the number of women suffering from ailments of the reproductive system would immediately fall and it is an apparatus which could, with benefit, be installed in every home.

Usually when alternate hot and cold Sitz baths are advised, the hot bath is used for four minutes and the cold bath for one minute, and the patient carries on in this way alternately for some ten to fifteen minutes. Cold Sitz baths are rather strenuous, but there is no other method which will give a quicker result in the loss of tone of the abdominal organs. They should, however, be of very short duration, say a few seconds to half a minute, and should be followed by a brisk reaction, leaving the patient feeling very fit and tingling with the rapidly circulating blood. If this reaction does not occur, the cold Sitz bath should be stopped until the vitality rises.

### The Cold Sponge

This is intended mainly as a tonic treatment which will invigorate the general skin circulation. It must also be of short duration, even during the summer months. In the winter time, it is advisable to fill a bath or basin with a little warm water and stand in it during the sponge down. It is best to use the bare hand, but a sponge, face cloth or friction brush may be used and the body should quickly be covered with water. Dry briskly by rubbing with the hands or rough towel and if there is a feeling of chilliness afterwards, take a drink of hot yeast extract.

# 5.
# What You can do about Headaches

DIETETIC ERRORS ARE responsible for most of the headaches of women and each person should study the diet, avoiding any food which appears allergic to that particular system. The first step is to write down a definite diet, hang it in the kitchen and adhere to these meals as strictly as possible. In this way, it is easy to find the food or liquid or combination of both which is causing the headache.

It is interesting to note that after Nature Cure has been followed for a month or two no digestive upset follows the eating of foods which were previously allergic. This is because a balanced diet changes the entire system and corrects the chemical unbalance which was formerly present.

## Bilious Headache

The pain is felt mainly on one side of the head and is usually accompanied by a nasty taste in the mouth. Some particular food is responsible for this type of headache. The tongue is usually furred and there is a heavy feeling in the liver area (near the lower right ribs). There may be constipation alternating with diarrhoea. Warm water should be taken in liberal quantities and the bowel cleansed by an enema or a mild vegetable laxative. Rest should be taken in a horizontal position, and the food suspected as the cause of the upset should be avoided in the future. Excessive fatty foods, two or more protein foods in combination, and chocolate or coffee should be suspect.

## Eye Headache

This headache often follows a period of eye strain such as close reading and the pain is usually above or behind the eyes. They feel hot, irritated and tired and there may be an acid discharge. In this condition the sight should be tested and the retina examined. Splashing cold water against the closed eyes will give relief.

## Frontal Headache

A headache which originates around the forehead, starts on rising and is persistently painful all morning, usually accompanies a kidney condition. The patient is inclined to vomit and to drowsiness and his sight may be affected. In all cases like this, the advice of a trained Nature Cure practitioner should be sought, because the blood pressure requires to be checked. A strict diet should be adhered to with a low protein content, and tea, coffee, aerated waters and synthetic fruit juices must be stopped. Waist compresses should be worn and regular exercises taken. Resting on the flat of the back should be avoided, because this adversely affects kidney drainage.

## Headache on Rising

Sleeping in a room where there is poor air circulation may cause this complaint, but kinking of the neck, resulting from pillows being too high, is a more common cause. In this latter state, rheumatic crystals will be found in or near the spine and the condition will be greatly relieved by hot and cold applications to the neck. Radiant heat and neck manipulation from a trained naturopath or osteopath is of great help.

Extreme irritability and a throbbing headache accompanied by fullness is frequently a sign that the blood pressure is above normal, although the symptoms arising from neck rheumatism are often very similar. A check of the blood pressure, however, makes the diagnosis clear.

If it is found that the blood pressure is above normal there is no need to panic because with careful treatment most of these conditions can be remedied. The way of life should be changed so that a rest is taken each afternoon and an occasional day in bed is obtained. The diet should be very simple and strictly vegetarian, being based on vegetables and fruit with very little starch or protein. Tea and coffee should be completely avoided and liquid should only be taken when there is actual thirst. Waist and neck compresses, as previously described, should be worn five nights a week.

It is not always possible to bring a very high blood pressure down to normal but in most cases the pressure can be controlled at a point which is not dangerous and headaches arising from it can thus be removed.

**Headache Due to Low Blood Pressure**

This type of headache is often caused by a mild brain anaemia following the loss of pressure and is usually relieved by the patient lying down. The condition is not *cured* by such methods and great patience and perseverance are required to raise the blood pressure once it has dropped to a very low level. Rest and exercise, especially deep breathing, are essential, and a diet rich in foods containing calcium and fluorine, is necessary. Liquids such as milk, yogurt, vegetable soup and fruit juices can be taken frequently. The waist compress can be worn five nights a week to retone the kidneys.

**Occipital Headache**

Sufferers from this type of headache, which is characterized by a dull continuous pain at the back of the head, should have their sight tested. Rheumatic crystals may also cause the pain when they are lying on or near the upper spinal nerves, and if these are present the pain can be relieved by radiant heat and the application of alternate hot and cold packs. A non-acid forming diet should be followed and massage obtained whenever possible. This latter treatment may be painful but any discomfort experienced will be worthwhile because this type of headache can be very wearing.

**Organic Headache**

One part of the head only is affected by this pain. It comes on at night and is so severe that it wakens the sufferer.

Frequently there is vomiting, which has no nausea or relation to food, and there is usually a feeling of drowsiness. Epileptic fits of a mild form are common and the pupils of the eyes become unequal in size. Professional advice should be sought immediately because these symptoms are very serious and may denote some destructive condition within the brain area.

**Sinus Headache**

This condition is usually caused by the suppression of a severe cold, resulting in catarrh congesting the facial sinuses around the eyes. Alternate hot and cold packs and steaming the face will give relief. The diet should be non-catarrhal and should be based on vegetables and fresh acid fruit. Milk in all forms should be avoided and starches taken in very small amounts.

The complete removal of headaches requires the studying of the body as a whole and treating it generally and locally. This means that our advice is not only to relieve pain but to tackle the underlying cause. This may have been present for years and usually has shown itself by slighter symptoms which were ignored or not even understood. Treat your body as a whole and you will obtain a measure of health which often seems impossible.

# 6.
# Facial Neuralgia

NEURALGIA OF ANY kind is one of the most painful ailments to which humans are prone but facial neuralgia can be most severe and many physicians believe that it is the most painful condition of all. The majority of sufferers are women, and there is reason to believe that the more sensitive system of the woman makes her more liable to this trouble.

Facial neuralgia is the term used when the pain is found in one or more branches of the facial nerve. Painful spots are above and below the eye, on the chin and near the ear. In addition to extreme sensitivity of the skin there is often swelling and discoloration and the sufferer is very careful to keep the part from being touched in any way.

There are many causes of this trouble. In a small percentage of cases it is a sign of brain tumour but generally it will be found that the nerve has been injured in some way and is being affected by pressure, anaemia, continual chilling of a part of the face or by an increase in the relative acidity of the blood.

If there is no alleviation night or day then the head should be X-rayed, as tumour formation may be the cause. If there is a history of injury to the head then again an X-ray is necessary to find out if there is nerve pressure. Often this is caused by a subluxation of the upper cervical bones and these should be examined by a competent Nature Cure practitioner. Subluxation is a very common cause of nerve pressure and is found in about seventy per cent of cases. Relative acidity of the blood is also a factor and the pressure on the nerve is then caused by rheumatic crystals which have formed in the area.

The facial nerve comes in close proximity to the teeth and if these are defective the mouth should be X-rayed. I once had a patient suffering from facial neuralgia without any apparent reason. An X-ray plate was taken of the mouth and the root of an old tooth lying high in the gum was discovered. Extraction of this root resulted in a complete cure.

Neuralgia usually comes on gradually. At first it is a transient attack of severe pain and for some time after it has gone the part feels tender and the sufferer experiences a desire to protect it from cold and touch. It is then that advice and treatment should be obtained as soon as possible because the condition rapidly becomes chronic. When this latter stage is reached the periods without pain become less frequent and the face assumes a certain contraction due to spasm of the muscles.

Treatment should be commenced during the acute stage with prolonged radiant heat. Lamps for this purpose can be obtained fairly cheaply but, failing this, the heat from an electric radiator should be applied to the part affected for some twenty minutes. The face must be protected from the cold. If possible, the neck bones should be examined for any subluxation by a Nature Cure practitioner because there is no home treatment for this common cause of the trouble. Neck manipulation is not a painful process and it is frequently followed by wonderful results.

If the blood is very 'acid' the prolonged milk diet is best, but if not entirely suitable it can be supplemented by vegetables, either steamed or raw, and vegetable soup. This diet will rapidly reduce the relative blood acidity and after the initial stages are over the diet should be mainly alkaline, using vegetable proteins in place of flesh foods, wholewheat bread instead of white, and honey instead of white sugar. Tea, coffee and aerated waters should be avoided, and the very acid fruits and fruit juices stopped temporarily. It must be stressed that when this trouble is due to food acid, the milk and vegetable diet will always prove the most beneficial.

# 7.
# Goitre

WHEN THEY READ of goitre, most people picture a swelling of the thyroid gland, but this complaint can be present without any swelling of the neck. Women are more prone to this serious upset which is caused by an over-production of thyroid secretion. It is a most difficult ailment to cure because it can be the final result of a breaking down of the glandular system. It is most important for the sufferer to seek advice as soon as the initial symptoms appear.

Goitre is more common in women who are overworked and who do not get sufficient rest and relaxation. The first symptoms are difficult to recognise because they are of very short duration, appearing merely as emotional upsets, and can pass almost unnoticed. Gradually these spells increase in length and there are other symptoms such as loss of power of concentration, depression and weeping and the sufferer appears to be very easily irritated. The approach of a nervous breakdown is often suspected.

The thyroid gland may swell but this has no relation to the severity of the ailment, because many serious cases have practically no visible swelling.

There is always a rapid though regular heart beat and any undue excitement increases this to a quick pulsation which may even be conveyed to the thyroid gland. There is, in most cases, a tremor of the hands and a feeling of extreme tiredness, together with a lack of power to make any real muscular effort. The eyes may incline to protrude, although this does not appear in all patients.

A most alarming symptom is the loss of weight which no treatment seems to check but which can persist until the lack of strength is extreme. All the above symptoms come on very gradually and that is why so many women do not complain until the trouble has reached serious proportions.

The periods in a woman's life when she is more likely to be affected in this manner are at puberty, during pregnancy, at the menopause or when there is any extra physical strain on the body.

Whenever it occurs it must not be assumed that it is a sudden flaring up, because goitre is not an abrupt derangement of a healthy system but a sign that there has been a gradual loss of health. In practically every instance the bowel is clogged and there has been a slow poisoning of the entire system over a period of years. It cannot be stressed too frequently that there is no sudden illness. Health always declines gradually and therefore regaining it must also be a gradual process. When the ailment arises in pregnancy however, it is often found that the toxic material causing the condition is coming from unhealthy gums or teeth or from some other unsuspected cause. Therefore, whenever a woman becomes pregnant she requires a complete examination with stress on the condition of the teeth, gums, tonsils, appendix and bowels.

Goitre is a serious complaint and quick results are essential to prevent irreparable harm but it should be remembered that great care must be exercised in the treatment of thyroid patients because of the unstable state of the sufferer. The excessive living rate and 'burning up' of the thyroid patient must be slowed and if this combustion is checked the chances of recovery are much increased.

Unfortunately, most sufferers have no knowledge of

food values and how correctly balanced meals containing plenty of health-giving salts can contribute largely to the curing of these ailments. In the first instance, there would be no glandular trouble if the body contained a sufficient supply of these vital health salts. Diet, therefore, is most important. For the first three days, nothing should be taken except fresh acid fruit with a glass of milk at each meal. After this the diet should be arranged as follows:

BREAKFAST

Fresh acid fruit such as apples, grapefruit, oranges, pears, grapes and one glass of whole milk.

MID-MORNING

One cup of yeast extract.

LUNCH

Vegetable soup to which agar extract has been added.

Protein such as cheese dish or egg dish or vegetarian savoury made from peas, beans, lentils or nuts.

Steamed or casseroled green and root vegetables.

One or two potatoes baked in their jackets.

Dessert: Fresh or dried fruit with occasionally a small helping of wholewheat steamed pudding or baked rice.

AFTERNOON

Milk or fruit juice.

EVENING MEAL

Vegetable soup.

Large raw salad containing any vegetable in season—lettuce, tomato, grated sprouts, cabbage, carrot, turnips, celery.

With this salad may be taken dried fruit such as dates or raisins or figs.

Toasted wholewheat bread, crisp bread, brown digestive

biscuit, etc.

Butter, honey.

SUPPER

Milk or fruit juice.

The appetite of the thyroid patient is usually very large and yet the weight reduction cannot be prevented from dropping for some time because, first of all, the heart beat must slow and the tremor vanish. Until this occurs there is incomplete assimilation of food, but as soon as this balance is restored, weight will slowly increase. To help the food to be absorbed, a narrow waist compress and, later, a neck compress should be worn five nights a week.

As weight is gained the almost constant hunger will gradually disappear. On no account should any stimulants be administered to create an appetite. Certain food and fluids are extremely injurious, such as white flour products, white sugar, flesh foods, fried or greasy foods, preserves, condiments, tea, coffee and alcohol. When the appetite has become normal it will determine the quantity of food required by that particular woman.

Nature Cure methods of healing do not include the taking of drugs of any description as these are foreign to the body and create irritation in the tissues. Iodine is undoubtedly most helpful in many cases, but it should be introduced in organic form, and all foods containing iodine should be taken liberally. These are asparagus, cabbage, carrots, garlic, onion, oats, pineapple, whole rice, agar extract, Carrageen moss, tomatoes, watercress and strawberries.

When the heart beat has been restored to normal and the weight has started to increase, the waist compress should be increased in width to ten inches and the neck compresses should also be worn. (Compresses explained in chapter on *Water Treatments*.)

Great care must be taken never to allow the body to

become exhausted and any irritation likely to cause emotional upset should be avoided. The cure of goitre is not a speedy one and there is often a recurrence of symptoms but these should gradually become less pronounced. Strict adherence to diet must be practised if complete cure is to be effected.

Always remember half the daily intake of food should consist of fresh fruit and vegetables, and the starch element should be confined to wholewheat products and potatoes (if possible the latter should be baked in their jackets). Potatoes are the most valuable form of starch. The protein (building and renewing) foods should be confined to egg, cheese, peas, beans, lentils and nuts. Milk and all flesh proteins must be avoided.

The diet outlined here should be strictly adhered to for a year, and the compresses on neck and waist applied for five consecutive nights a week for two months and discontinued for one month. Water treatments should be taken to increase skin elimination. Apply a warm soapy sponge to the entire body before retiring and a cold sponge on rising. The latter should be continued only if there is a good reaction; if this is experienced, the overstraining of the other eliminating organs will be diminished.

Hot baths are weakening and tend to spoil the skin action and are therefore not advised. It is most important that the bowels are kept working efficiently so there is no more danger of a toxic condition of the blood arising from that source.

The treatment outlined above will not fail to improve the condition, provided the sufferer perseveres and understands that complete health can only be regained slowly.

The emotional aspect must be studied and every effort made to prevent emotional stress. For some considerable time there will be slight recurrence of this extremely nervous complaint, but the attacks will become less severe and of shorter duration as the treatment progresses. If, however, they are too numerous and of an exceedingly serious nature, a trained Naturopath should be consulted. In all these treatments there must be no lessening of the woman's efforts to help herself because success can only be attained by assiduous effort.

# 8.
# Breast Troubles

FEW BREAST TROUBLES are actually malignant and the wise woman seeks professional advice as soon as any peculiarity of the breast structure is discovered. In many cases Nature Cure treatment is very effective and even when recourse to surgery is necessary our methods do much to retone the part and prevent the spread of the trouble.

### Heaviness of the Breast Before Menstruation

Many women become concerned about this symptom thinking it may be an indication of some serious complaint. This peculiar heavy feeling is due to over-activity of the ovaries and the commencement of the menstrual flow usually brings relief and gradually the breasts become of normal size. Heaviness of the breast after childbirth, especially if the child is not breast fed, is also common. In such cases it is usual to find that the breast ducts are choked and small nodules can be felt. These are really harmless and can be removed by skilled massage and by bathing the breasts with alternate hot and cold water. This is a very safe application and ideal for stimulating the circulation, but some time may elapse before the breast is completely clear.

### Breast Abscess

An abscess of the breast is a most painful condition. It occurs most commonly in nursing mothers, especially when there is lowered health. The symptoms can be constitutional and there may be malaise, fever and general upset. The part becomes inflamed and enlarges with considerable discomfort and pain, and a red area shows where the abscess is pointing. Immediately these symptoms are noticed the woman should be fasted and whenever possible the bowel cleansed by a warm water enema. The diet should consist of fruit and fruit juices only and all other food stopped. Milk in particular should be avoided. Local treatment should consist of applying wet cold cloths over the part, changing them very frequently. In this way the abscess may soften and burst without any pain and then it should be encouraged to discharge by compressing until every sign of inflammation or pus have gone. I have treated a number of abscesses in this way with remarkably successful results.

Not all abscesses can be controlled by cold water compressing and still continue to 'point' but I prefer to allow them to rupture of their own accord; in any case, hot applications should not be used until the very last minute. The alternate hot and cold pack is a much better way of treating the 'pointing' abscess than by poulticing. Once the abscess has burst the cold pack should be worn over the wound and continued until the part is perfectly drained. Abscess formation is a sign that the body is below par and steps should be taken to ensure better health by a Nature Cure diet.

### Inflammation of the Breast

Inflammation of the breast often occurs at puberty and during the menopause. There is a general swelling of the breast substance and this is followed by considerable discomfort. Pains often radiate to the arm-pit and down the arm.

Whenever the condition is severe the girl or woman should be fasted and the breast should be bathed frequently with alternate hot and cold water. Between times the breast should be bandaged with cotton wool after massaging gently with warm olive oil. If the condition is prolonged the waist compress should be worn combined with a local breast compress. The inflamed breast should always be supported.

### Large Breasts

Exceedingly large breasts cause much discomfort. They are occasionally the result of glandular upset but are often connected with general obesity. In the latter case a reducing diet is necessary and it will be found that the breasts will become smaller as the body becomes thinner. To increase the circulation, sponge frequently with cold water and do the breast exercises explained at the end of this chapter. Massage by a skilled practitioner is also useful in increasing drainage. The diet should be a 'dry' one, that is, fluid must be reduced as much as possible and plenty of fruit and vegetables eaten.

### Small Breasts

Small and very poorly developed breasts in a woman otherwise normally developed are unnatural. I have had several cases of this kind and have found they can be improved by careful treatment. First of all I believe in a diet with plenty of fluid, especially milk, but of course always on balanced Nature Cure lines. An oil massage using warm olive oil or nut oil is also most helpful, but it should be conducted by a practitioner as massage of the breasts by an unskilled person can be harmful. Finally the breast exercises should be practised assiduously and then I am sure than an improvement in development will follow.

**Cyst in the Breast**

This appears as a small lump and usually causes great alarm because it is frequently suspected to be something very serious. The most common cause is a previous incorrectly drained abscess but poor circulation in any form will ultimately bring about the formation of these cysts. In any cause, professional advice should be sought immediately and once it is diagnosed as a simple cyst with no adhesions to the chest wall or formation of thickening in the armpit glands, then it can be treated by natural methods.

The general aim is the disposal of the cyst but here a word of warning is necessary. The person should not attempt to MASSAGE it away as this can be most harmful. Cysts should not be handled in any way. The best method is to treat the whole body in an effort to bring about increased drainage. A day or two on fresh acid fruit is the ideal start to the treatment because nothing increases the activity of the lymphatic (drainage) system more than fruit fast. After this the food should be arranged on the lines already outlined in the chapter on diet but milk in any form should be avoided.

Cold packs should be used locally over the cyst and a waist compress should be worn. The breast exercises should be practised carefully. A quick result cannot be expected but these methods will result in a gradual reduction of the cyst. At present I am treating a patient who had one large cyst in each breast and she had made a rapid recovery on fruit fasting and compressing without any other treatment. The value of fresh acid fruit cannot be stressed too much in this condition.

**Cancer**

Breast cancer is difficult to diagnose but it shows a swelling which, when pressed against the chest wall, tends to become more prominent and which has adhesions to the surrounding structure, making it practically immovable. It arises, like every other form of cancer as a result of debris within the body piling up until it must be deposited in a part of weakened drainage. Wrong habits of living and the constant suppression of the eliminating reactions of the body are mainly responsible.

Under the Pharmacy and Drugs Act, 1941, it is illegal for anyone to 'advertise' treatment for certain diseases, including cancer. In any case, such conditions are outside the scope of a book of this nature.

## Breast Exercises

EXERCISE ONE: Stand erect with hands clenched. Hold them at shoulder level in front of the body, also keeping the elbows high. Now press the clenched fists together when a strain will be felt in the chest and the breasts will rise. Press. Relax. Continue in this fashion until tired. This exercise drains the breasts and is ideal when there is sagging of the muscles of the glands.

EXERCISE TWO: Same position as Exercise One, but with the fingers of one hand gripped in the fingers of the other. Pull the right hand round towards the right side and resist as much as possible with the left hand. Then pull with the left hand and resist with the right. This is a strong exercise which lifts and drains the breasts.

EXERCISE THREE: Stand erect with the arms by the side. Now swing the right arm forward and upward and backward, completing the full circle. Continue in this way for some twenty swings. Then do the same movement with the left arm. This exercise retones the muscles of the chest wall and increases tissue drainage.

# 9. Migraine

IN ALMOST EVERY case the headache is one-sided and most often just over the eye. There may be a constant throbbing and even after the bout has passed a peculiar feeling of dullness persists for several days. Other sufferers feel completely clear as soon as the attack is over, and there seem to be no after-effects.

Many women suffering from this complaint find that exposure to any light becomes unbearable, and so complete rest in a darkened room is essential. In other cases the headache is actually preceded by a visual disturbance in which the sufferer experiences a series of bright flashes in the field of vision. This flashing becomes very intense as the headache comes on and is commonly followed by nausea and vomiting.

It may be much more of a general upset, however, and there may be a tingling of the arms and hands. It has been known for the speech to become disturbed immediately prior to the actual attacks. The bladder may become irritated and a large quantity of urine voided. This latter type of migraine is not so common but there are certain women who suffer from these exceedingly distressing symptoms. There is usually some warning a few days before the attack, such as a feeling of tiredness, lack of appetite or nausea. When this warning occurs it will often be found that a complete fast will prevent an attack.

The usual treatment for migraine is some form of drug and this eases the pain temporarily. There can, however, be no real cure along these lines.

Migraine can arise as a result of an overworked nervous system or from physical exhaustion. There are more common causes, however, such as the taking of allergic foods or fluids, clogged condition of the bowel, digestive upset or liver congestion. In a great number of cases the cause is not easily discovered. The taking of certain foods and their effects must be carefully studied to discover if there is an allergy, and the sufferer from migraine must pay particular attention to the bowel to ensure elimination. It is often helpful to have the eyes tested by a competent oculist because there may be an error of refraction.

After fasting, the sufferer would be well advised to eat only fresh fruit for several days. Then a balanced Nature Cure diet should be adopted and carefully followed. This diet must be continued for a long time because this trouble is difficult to eradicate if the cause is in the digestive system.

**Bone Displacement**

Recent experiments have proved that almost every sufferer from migraine has a neck lesion and very often the first three upper spinal bones are displaced. In mild cases this dislocation can be corrected by the application of alternate hot and cold packs to the neck and by practising relaxation exercises. If, however, there is a severe dislocation. manipulation is necessary and a trained naturopath or osteopath should be consulted. Often a few manipulations result in a complete removal of the migraine attack.

This correction of the small cervical bones is quite painless, and no amount of other treatment will cure the migraine if a mechanical fault such as subluxation is at the root of the trouble.

# 10.
# Menstrual Difficulties

THE MENSTRUAL FLOW is a provision of nature to cleanse the inner surfaces of the womb and enable reproduction to take place normally. The flow generally commences about the fourteenth year and continues for some thirty years. It normally lasts about four days and has a rhythm of some twenty-eight days, but this varies considerably and regularity is the most important factor. Normal menstruation should be practically painless and much of the trouble experienced by women at this time is due to the unnatural methods of eating and exercising. The woman who follows a Nature Cure way of life very often finds that all her menstrual difficulties clear up as the body becomes healthier.

## Painful Menstruation

Pain starting two or three days before the flow usually shows that the ovaries are not functioning properly. This is a glandular misfunction and careful dieting will usually put matters right. For local treatment, hot Sitz baths on alternate nights for a week before the period is due will often bring about a cure. Between periods the cold Sitz baths will increase the tone of the ovaries. If pain still occurs after this treatment has been tried, then the services of a trained naturopath should be obtained because manipulative treatment is often curative. It usually consists of adjusting the lower thoracic and lumbar vertebrae and frequently has marvellous results.

Pain immediately before the flow commences is indicative of uterine flexion, which means that the position of the womb is abnormal. A professional examination is required to find how the womb is lying and then a series of exercises can be arranged whereby correction is maintained. Uterine flexion often occurs in women who are so thin that they have lost internal fat and the ligament on which the womb is suspended has lost tone. General treatment along the dietetic lines is required in addition to the exercises. Twisting of the womb forward usually means that frequency of the bladder results and when the womb falls backwards, then the bowel function is disturbed. Inclined-board exercises are very beneficial in both conditions, but professional advice is always required.

When the pain occurs during menstruation it usually means that the womb itself is inflamed. There are several forms of this but, generally speaking, they can all be aided by careful attention to diet, by hot Sitz baths taken just before the period is due and cold Sitz baths between the period times. Pain-relieving drugs are not a real cure and cannot be advised because they only make the trouble more chronic. Sun-ray and radiant heat treatment is very beneficial in many cases and can be thoroughly recommended. Whenever possible, naturopathic manipulative movement will do much to increase the circulation around the reproductive organs.

### Stoppage of Menstruation

Stoppage of menstruation is natural during pregnancy and at the menopause, but abnormal at any other time. Certainly there are some women who have very infrequent periods but this seems to be peculiar to their particular type and cannot be termed a true stoppage. If, however, the periods have been quite regular for a number of years and then suddenly stop or the cycle becomes frequently interrupted and there has been no actual causative factor, then one of the following conditions may be present:

### Tuberculosis

There is usually loss of weight, night sweats and general listlessness, and if these are noticed, a trained practitioner should be consulted immediately because such a trouble is not within the sphere of home treatment. Young girls most frequently suffer from this condition, which in many cases is transient and can be corrected by professional care.

### Excessive Mental and Emotional Strain

If the patient has a history of this upset, removal of the cause and a careful regime of rest and building up along Nature Cure lines will result in a return of normal menstruation, although this may be delayed several months until the body is strong enough to cleanse the womb. Stoppage of menstruation in these cases is the body's effort to conserve energy.

### Chill

Menstruation frequently stops as the result of a chill just before the period is due. Hot Sitz baths may bring it on again but it is likely that the period will be missed and the next one more profuse.

Before any period commences, special attention should be paid to the feet and legs because if they become very cold the blood circulation through the womb is retarded. It is a very good plan to immerse the feet in hot water for ten minutes if it is felt that they are too cold.

### Displacement

There may be some twisting of the womb and surrounding organs. This condition frequently causes disturbed menstrual function and can be the result of an accident or due to a great loss of fat after a debilitating illness. Either the broad ligament sags or the womb falls forward or backward and the resulting kinking impairs the blood flow.

## Anaemia

This is the most common cause of irregular menstruation and is frequently found in young girls, when the condition is known as *chlorosis.*

Rest is absolutely essential and the patient should be kept in bed for one or two weeks to ensure that the body is allowed to regain its strength.

All exercise should be stopped except a certain amount of deep breathing and slow walking. A course of artificial sunlight treatment should be obtained whenever possible. The skin should be bathed with warm soapy water each morning followed by a short cold sponge and friction rub. The entire body should be sponged with warm soapy water each night, but hot baths should be avoided. Occasionally a warm, not hot, Sitz bath should be taken.

The most common error in the treatment of anaemia is overfeeding. Surely, if rest is essential, then resting the digestive tract is just as important and much better results are obtained by having a few weeks on restricted diet, such as the following:

ON RISING

Glass of warm water should be sipped.

BREAKFAST

1. Fresh acid fruit and whole milk (in any quantity)

or

2. Bran with dried fruit (soaked and then simmered). Wholewheat bread. Milk, or yeast extract.

or

3. Fresh egg, lightly poached or boiled
   Milk and fruit

LUNCH

Vegetable, tomato or lentil soup.

Cheese pudding or egg dish or nut dish or vegetarian dish made from peas, beans and lentils.

Steamed vegetables and baked or steamed potatoes.
Dessert: Fruit or milk.

EVENING MEAL
Soup
Raw vegetable salad containing all vegetables and fruit in season with wholewheat bread or toast or any kind of crisp bread.
Butter, honey.

SUPPER
Fruit or milk

No food should be taken between meals.

It should be realized that stoppage of menstruation in the case of the anaemic person means the blood has been considerably weakened, and a quick return of the menstrual flow cannot be expected. Two to four months may pass without menstruation while the body is being built up, but this need cause no worry if it is evident that the patient is making physical progress. Once the blood is of good quality and quantity then the flow will again function normally.

## Excessive Menstruation

Profuse menstrual flow is common in certain women and usually denotes a blood deficiency, frequently of blood calcium, although there are also cases of prolonged and profuse uterine bleeding which are nature's method of ridding the blood of impurities. It may, however, be an indication of a very serious condition and the advice of a practitioner should be obtained as quickly as possible, especially if the patient is at the menopausal stage. Every effort should be made to stop this excessive bleeding by natural methods before resorting to the use of drugs.

It is essential to keep the patient absolutely quiet and

confined to bed, the bottom of which should be raised four or five inches. If the bleeding is very bad, a gauze plug may be inserted into the vagina as a temporary measure, as many women become exceedingly alarmed and this tends to aggravate the condition.

For the first few days the diet should consist only of milk and raw vegetables. No stimulants should be taken as they tend to increase the flow.

When the bleeding has stopped, great care must be taken to avoid over-exercising or straining the body in any manner. For several weeks all movements should be as gentle as possible.

A full Nature Cure diet should then be adopted using fresh raw vegetable salads twice daily. Artificial sunlight, peritoneal douches, and abdominal exercises to tone the muscles are most beneficial at this point. Cold Sitz baths of very short duration are also extremely helpful provided the patient has a good reaction.

Excessive uterine bleeding after the menopause may be a symptom of a serious trouble and professional advice should be sought immediately the condition occurs.

# 11. The Menopause

THE MENOPAUSAL CHANGE is not a disease but a perfectly normal event which occurs in women between the ages of forty and fifty. In a really healthy person it takes place without any symptoms, and in many women the only sign that it has taken place is the cessation of the periods. Internally, of course, the glandular secretions have stopped and as a result of this the nervous system should become more stable with resultant poise and relaxation.

When annoying and disagreeable symptoms appear at the customary menopausal time it means either that the woman is not prepared emotionally for the change or that she is in poor physical condition.

## Emotions

At this time many women feel that they are becoming old and are well past their full physical zenith. This is absolute nonsense, and it should be stressed that in many native races, women find that their capacity for heavy physical tasks increases after menopause and they often return to the work at which they were employed during their teens.

Again, many childless married women regret the passing of the possibility of their having a child. It should be appreciated that the real survival of the race depends on women having a family while they themselves are physically fit, active and able to deal successfully with the difficult task of bringing up their children. Unmarried women, on the other hand, may feel that the menopause means that their last chance of having children is lost and that life has become pointless. Life in middle age can be anything but useless and, indeed, in most cases it can be made much more rewarding that at any other time.

Other women feel that the menopause brings a cessation of sexual pleasure. Actually there need be no decrease in sexual vigour or enjoyment. Deeper understanding should mean that the embrace can be still enjoyed by both partners, and this often leads to a deeper sympathy and an understanding of marriage which was hitherto lacking. This point should be fully understood because many women tend to shun their husbands at this time and thus sow the seeds of much friction. Sexual activity after the menopause is not wrong; indeed, it is possible for a women at any age to enjoy sex just as deeply as she did in her youth.

The change of life usually brings a change of personality; most women tend to become more reasonable and sympathetic towards the foibles of youth and this leads to a contentment and relaxation which are really essential to full health. The menopause marks not the end of youth but the beginning of a new way of life.

**Physical Changes**

Most women enter middle age without real physical preparation. The period, in addition to having a sexual function, also acts as a means of elimination of impurity and when this is lost the blood-stream may become clogged so that symptoms of ill-health begin to appear. The wise woman, in her thirties, takes steps to build up her eliminative capacity before the menstrual flow ceases and the following measures will ensure success in this respect.

We have four eliminative organs—the skin, the kidneys, the lungs and the bowel, and, when a balanced diet is taken, these organs, working correctly, are capable of keeping the blood-stream pure.

**The Skin**

This tissue should never be over-clad, and so light but warm underwear should be worn. Too many hot baths are unnecessary, and warm, soapy, cleansing rubs are more healthful, especially if they are followed by a quick, cold sponge down and a brisk friction rub. Generally speaking, sun-lamp treatment is good for the skin, especially during the winter months, but as much sun stimulation as possible should be gained during the summer.

**The Kidneys**

Excessive amounts of tea, coffee and alcoholic drinks do great harm to the kidneys, and these alone can make the physical symptoms of the menopause more irritating and severe. Reduce these liquids very severely and take clear vegetable soup and other vegetable drinks, pressed vegetable and fruit juice, and plenty of water when actually thirsty.

### Breathing and the Lungs

In practice, it is the exception rather than the rule to find a woman in middle life who breathes properly. The best plan is to visit a competent Nature Cure practitioner for advice or to take a course of deep breathing from a local physical training instructor. This pays wonderful dividends.

### The Bowels

A diet reform regimen in itself ensures proper bowel action because it is largely eliminative. Avoid white bread and white sugar, and take only a small amount of protein each day, eliminating excessive amounts of meat and fish and having no more that three eggs weekly. Large amounts of salads and fruits form the basis of a healthful dietary. Such a régime will help greatly to reduce any impurity which may have been built up in the body.

Finally, the middle-aged woman should have an interest in life. An active pursuit, such as painting, gardening or social work, should be studied and followed because such activities lead to the sedation and relaxation which are necessary to enable one to deal with life's problems.

# 12. Leucorrhoea

THIS CATARRHAL DISCHARGE from the vagina is one of the most common of women's ailments and one about which they rarely seek advice until it is chronic and then difficult to cure.

In certain women there is a tendency to vaginal discharge immediately before the menstrual flow starts and it is not apparent at any other time, It is usually very slight and lasts only a few days. On the other hand, there are women who have an almost uninterrupted heavy catarrhal flow and this condition is most difficult to clear up. Scrupulous cleanlinesss of the vagina is essential and if there is going to be a real cure, a diet of non-catarrhal forming foods must be strictly adhered to.

In acute cases this discharge is the result of chill by getting wet feet or sitting on a damp seat. Chilling causes inflammation of the womb and vaginal membranes and the resulting excretion may be extremely heavy.

Other common causes are womb displacement and impurities in the body cavity and catarrhal reproductive tissues. The discharge always tends to become more troublesome in women who are in occupations where they are standing for long periods.

Generally the sufferers complain of tiredness and a dragging sensation in the abdomen. Hot Sitz baths are very beneficial and should be taken nightly. The hips should be immersed in hot water for ten minutes, after which the patient should go to bed immediately to avoid all risk of chilling.

Douching is the most effective method of cleansing the vagina but warm water only should be used. All disinfectants should be avoided as they have a suppressive action and can eventually lead to much more serious trouble. The presence of leucorrhoea is definitely an indication of a catarrhal condition and every effort should be made to encourage the body to eliminate its impurity. This can never be accomplished by using disinfectants.

It is surprising to find that a great many women regard the douche as something to be avoided at all times. To use it too frequently where there is no discharge is not good treatment, but occasionally it is advisable, I think, to use this method in order to ensure complete vaginal cleanliness.

The vaginal douche is used in the following manner. Put two pints of warm water in the douche can and hang at a level of about three feet above the body. This will prevent the water entering the vagina with too great a force and could be harmful. The patient should lie with the hips raised slightly above the level of the body and the nozzle should be oiled or rubbed with a little vaseline and inserted slowly into the vagina. The flow can be regulated by the small valve at the nozzle. In severe leucorrhoea, this douche should be taken nightly.

If the condition is very obstinate a warm water douche preceded by a hot Sitz bath will be found most helpful, and if the patient has a good reaction to cold water applications, a cold Sitz bath of one minute's duration may be taken first thing in the morning.

As the condition is not merely the outcome of one organ being affected, but the result of a system completely choked and impure, a full Nature Cure régime should be adopted.

The cold water compress is most beneficial in the treatment of this complaint and should be worn five nights a week. The entire body should be sponged once a day, preferably on rising, with cold water followed by a vigorous friction rub. Correct diet is necessary and one based on the following lines will be most helpful:

ON RISING

Glass of orange or lemon juice in hot water.

BREAKFAST

Fresh acid fruit only. This includes apples, oranges, pears, grapefruit, lemons, all berries, plums, etc. Fruit juice may also be taken.

LUNCH

Vegetable soup.

Cheese pudding or egg dish or vegetarian savoury with conservatively cooked vegetables and baked or steamed potatoes.

Dessert: fresh or dried fruit.

EVENING MEAL

Vegetable soup.

Large salad using every kind of vegetable in season, also dates, figs, raisins, pineapple, grated pear, apple, etc.

Small amount of starch in the form of wholewheat products or any other crisp bread or brown digestive biscuit. Butter.

Yeast extract if there is actual thirst.

SUPPER

Fruit only.

Fresh fruit only should be taken between meals. All forms of white flour, white sugar (use honey) fried and greasy foods, condiments, preserves, milk, tea and coffee, should be avoided.

If the above methods are practised vigorously, this troublesome complaint can generally be cured. There may, however, be cases where the trouble is exceedingly obstinate and if so the services of a Nature Cure practitioner are required for spinal manipulation and the application of infra-red rays.

If leucorrhoea is very profuse, the constant flow of this acid catarrhal discharge may cause great discomfort to the patient by its corroding action on the vaginal walls. A gauze pack dipped into a paste made from Slippery Elm and cold water and inserted into the vagina for short periods will prove most soothing. If actual ulceration of the vagina occurs a practitioner should be consulted.

# 13.
# Sterility

IN SPITE OF the latest scientific findings about the various blood groups, sterility still ranks high as a reason for unhappy marriage. The most common cause is malformation or sagging of the womb and for this surgical treatment is often necessary. Collapse of the Fallopian tubes is another factor and here methods of inflation are useful. It would seem therefore that sterility comes largely within the province of the surgeon, but this is not always the case and Nature Cure methods have often proved successful when everything else has failed.

Sterility is very frequently caused by poor circulation, lowered muscular tone and catarrhal conditions of the reproductive system. But before we discuss these I wish to pause for a moment and examine the mechanics of conception. By doing so we can gain a knowledge of how to direct our treatment.

The male sperms are shed into the vagina during intercourse and at the very same time an alkaline fluid is secreted from the vaginal walls. Only when this fluid is present are the mobile sperms able to pass up the womb and through the Fallopian tubes to fertilize the female egg. If there is a break in this succession of events then sterility is certain and we must look for weak spots.

Two factors are necessary to ensure there is a normal secretion of the alkaline fluid. The first is that the nerve supply to the vaginal ducts must be perfect and this is where the very nervous woman fails and sterility results. In such cases the nervous system must be built up by adequate rest, relaxation, infrequent intercourse, and a diet based on the one described in the previous chapter. It is wonderful how such treatment will result in a relaxation of the tense nervous system.

The second point is that the fluid flowing from the vaginal walls must be of an alkaline nature. If this is not so then the sperms are destroyed by the acidic fluid which is usually present in the vaginal canal and womb. To ensure that the fluid which flows during intercourse is alkaline, it is necessary to balance the diet by introducing a large amount of vegetables (especially raw) and fruit and reduce all demineralized and acid-forming foods. The diet already outlined is arranged on this basis and should be carefully followed by any woman who appears to be infertile.

During their actual passage through the womb and Fallopian tubes the sperms are again subjected to other attacks. They are easily destroyed by any acid substance and the most common in these organs is the acid discharge known as leucorrhoea. If this discharge is constant, then the chances of fertilization are very much reduced.

Leucorrhoea is difficult to cure, but dieting enters largely into its treatment, which is described in another part of this book.

When the sperms reach the womb they should pass easily upwards into the openings of the Fallopian tubes on either side. If, however, the womb is not lying naturally then the path of the sperms becomes difficult. There are several causes of the womb being out of position and the most common is sagging of the broad ligament which supports it. This often arises when the woman suddenly loses abdominal fat and here injudicious slimming is an important factor. The woman who is overweight should only slim under professional advice because this vital abdominal fat must not be lost or prolapse takes place. Of course, there are other causes of loss of abdominal fat such as poor food, nervous conditions affecting the swallowing, acidic troubles of the stomach and duodenum, colitis of the bowel and so on. If, however, a large amount of abdominal fat is lost then displacement of the womb is common and sterility may result.

The womb can also be displaced as the result of an accident such as a heavy weight falling on the back, a severe fall or as a result of lifting too heavy objects.

It is usually possible to tell when the womb is out of position because there is often a severe dragging pain in the back. There are also symptoms at menstruation during which the bladder and the lower bowel become abnormal in some way. When it is felt that there has been some change in the womb position, professional naturopathic advice should be sought. In most cases the cure lies in exercising on the inclined board plus compressing and Sitz baths, and by these measures many women have corrected the condition.

When the Fallopian tubes have collapsed the condition is difficult to diagnose and correct, and when it is found, some method of inflation of these tubes is usually necessary. Often only one tube is affected and there are cases of women becoming pregnant if they sleep on their other side.

If there is pain three days before the period this usually means there is some inflammation of the ovaries and it is common to suppose that this is caused by a catarrhal conditon of the Fallopian tubes. Then alternate hot and cold Sitz baths should be used and the diet should be a non-catarrhal one built on the following lines:

BREAKFAST

Fruit of any kind and fruit juice.

LUNCH

Vegetable soup.

Meat or steamed or baked fish or cheese dish or vegetarian savoury with steamed vegetables and one or two baked potatoes.

Dessert: Fruit only.

EVENING MEAL

Salad with wholewheat bread or crisp bread or brown fruit cake.
Butter, honey.

Of course there are many other causes of sterility. Many women never actually have intercourse due to some malformation of the vagina. This can often be corrected by surgery as also can a thickened hymen which will not rupture. Fibroid tumours of the womb are another common cause. When soft, these tumours can be removed by strict Nature Cure methods, but when they are very hard and enlarging rapidly, then I think surgery is indicated.

# 14.

# Cystitis

(*Inflammation of the bladder*)

---

ACUTE CYSTITIS IS a most common complaint in women and usually follows chilling of the feet and legs. Prolonged retention of urine or gravel in the bladder may be the actual cause. The pain is mainly between the legs and over the bladder region and may extend up to and round the kidney area. There is general malaise, fever and frequent micturition with cloudiness of the urine. Bleeding can also occur and this usually distresses the patient very much, but it is not of great significance.

The main treatment consists of rest and heat. The hips and lower abdomen should be immersed in hot water as described under Sitz Baths in the chapter on water treatments, and several of these baths are needed during the acute stage. Relief can also be obtained by the application of hot cloths over the bladder area. Barley water, parsley tea or buttermilk should be taken in quantity during this period if the urine is greatly thickened, but should gradually be reduced when this disagreeable symptom disappears.

When the condition is chronic, the fluid in the diet should be kept at moderate proportions, but all tea, coffee, aerated waters, wines, spirits and alcohol should be strictly avoided. Limit the fluid to water, milk, buttermilk, yeast extract, barley water or parsley tea, and take only enough to keep the urine in a free-flowing state. I think the 'dry' diet, which is frequently advised in Nature Cure, is unsuitable for people having this condition.

Proteins are also dangerous irritants in cystitis and should be reduced in quantity until only one is taken daily. Choose from peas, beans, lentils, eggs, cheese, milk and nuts. Avoid flesh proteins completely. This will seem a great hardship to many people but reduction of protein will result in considerable abatement of the irritation.

In chronic cases, attention must be paid to retoning the system, because a loss of muscular power in the bladder wall is always present. This takes time and patience and it may be six months before elderly patients feel the benefit of the treatment.

It is essential that the call of nature is never unduly delayed and the bladder is always completely emptied. Retention of urine, especially if it is very acid, irritates the bladder wall and causes inflammation, making the condition most difficult to cure.

Liquids should be strictly limited to those mentioned above and should only be taken when there is actual thirst or when the urine is much thickened. The proteins also must be limited.

During warm weather, the best water treatment to use is

cold sponging or spraying of the bladder area and between the legs. This should be done twice daily or even more frequently but it must be performed quickly and there should be a good reaction. A feeling of warmth in the parts should occur after a few minutes; if this reaction is not obtained, the treatment is too severe or too protracted.

If the patient is fairly vital and there are no high blood pressure or serious heart complications, the quick cold Sitz bath is easily the most tonic treatment. This need only last a few seconds and it also should be accompanied by a feeling of well-being if the desired reaction is obtained.

This method should be aided by side-bending and body rolling exercises and, if need be, by manipulative treatment to the lower spine, because there is very commonly some displacement. If the foregoing treatment is followed carefully and there is no result, spinal manipulation should always be obtained.

The general Nature Cure diet mentioned at the beginning of this book is necessary to introduce the mineral salts needed to control the acidity of the urine.

# 15. Obesity

CERTAIN WOMEN ARE naturally stout and, because their girth comes from muscle, they are perfectly healthy and remain so until their muscles lose tone. This is not the type of person I am writing about however, but rather the type of woman who has gradually put on layer upon layer of fat until the entire musculature of the body has become fatty and out of tone, and whose abdomen is huge and prolapsed. This condition is not only very disfiguring, but is also extremely serious because the excessive fat spreads from the muscles inward until it affects the vital organs such as the liver, heart and kidneys.

Once this stage is reached the condition becomes dangerous to life and it is no exaggeration to say that the person who is below normal weight after forty has a much greater chance of a longer and healthier life than the person who is even a few pounds overweight.

Obesity, then, should be regarded as a disease and the cause always should be sought. Most people blame some disfunction of the glandular system, but decreased physical activity and overeating will account for ninety per cent of the cases of obesity. Certainly glandular trouble does come into the picture, but no so frequently as people think and the general Nature Cure methods will deal adequately even with this cause.

Young girls try reducing without sufficient knowledge of the subject and over the past few years many have reduced past the normal. In so doing they weaken their general strength and run the risk of tuberculosis. This, of course, had led to many authorities stressing the dangers of rigid dieting and I must add my own warning. Before any reducing is attempted the general health state should be examined and it is best to visit a registered Nature Cure practitioner for guidance in this matter. It is generally safe to diet if it is really felt that the weight is excessive, although the physical condition does not seem to be much impaired.

Do not attempt to bring down the weight rapidly because the blood pressure and other factors may be quickly upset and then more harm than good will result. Aim at a weight loss of a pound or two each week and try not to exceed this. If you find the loss is rapid and amounts to five or six pounds weekly, then you are being too vigorous and more food and liquid should be taken. Weight comes down quite rapidly at the beginning, so diet rather moderately to start with and become more rigid as the rate of loss slows down. Often there seems to be a stage when the weight remains the same for a week or two. Do not be dismayed at this turn of events but continue with your dieting and gradually the weight loss will again appreciate.

Before any dieting is attempted, exercise should be increased. Move around the house more quickly. Walk instead of taking the bus, and try to get a brisk walk each day even if it is a very short distance. This brings about an increase in the circulation and will slim the body even if it does not reduce the weight. A quicker circulation is essential to weight reducing because the impurities have to be conveyed to the eliminating organs.

Another good way of increasing the circulation is to use cold water on the skin. Have the cold rub each morning. Better still, if you are fairly fit, have a cold spray or quick cold bath. These cause an intense coldness on the skin and bring about a rapid flow of blood, and many impurities are removed by the increased lymphatic flow. Many people, of course, cannot take such vigorous treatment and they should content themselves with the quick cold rub even if it is taken after a cleansing warm bath.

The majority of women drink too much fluid and this increases their weight by filling the tissues with liquid and bringing about a water-logged condition. A certain quantity of fluid is required by the body each day but this is mainly obtained from fruit and vegetables. As this is pure distilled water, it is actually the best source of liquid. Tea, coffee, cocoa and aerated waters are all fluids which are not required by the body. They are not foods but could be termed mild poisons and certainly do create the conditions which lead to obesity. So the third point is the reducing of the amount of fluid intake, only drinking water, fruit juices and vegetable soup when there is actual thirst. This stoppage of fluid will often work wonders and

I know many women who have obtained a perfect weight and figure by these measures alone.

## The First Change

The changing of the diet itself should be a gradual process. Enter into dieting rather slowly and you will find that no great upset follows. The breakfast meal should be the first to be altered. It will usually be found that the fresh acid fruit is the best type of breakfast for the person attempting to reduce. Choose from apples, oranges, pears, plums, grapefruit, grapes, strawberries and all such berries. There is no limit to quantity and any kind of mixture may be taken although each person will soon find out the fruits which are most agreeable. If desired, especially during the winter months, soaked and simmered prunes, figs, raisins and apricots may be taken in small quantity. These give some bulk to the fruit breakfast because they are inclined to be of a sugar-starch nature. Fluid should also be avoided with the fruit diet, but many people feel they need something hot to drink with such a meal and on cold days a glass of lemon or orange juice and hot water may be taken. No other food or liquid should be included at this meal.

It is much better to establish the fruit breakfast before correcting another meal, so at least a week should elapse before there are any more changes. During this time the results of the fruit breakfast can be studied and fruit which proves indigestible can be omitted from the diet. Most people feel unsatisfied after such a breakfast and there will be a desire for solid food during the morning. This feeling should be resisted and will soon pass. A slight weight loss should be noted after one week.

## The Second Change

Usually soup is taken at the midday meal, but this will naturally be stopped because of the required dryness of the diet. Due to the lack of fluid it is likely that many people will become constipated. This will gradually correct itself but a few weeks may naturally elapse before normal bowel action is achieved. It is better therefore, to stop food which decays in the intestine if constipation is present, and this includes all flesh foods and fish. Indeed, if real health is to be gained and maintained, these can be dispensed with altogether.

The second meal (the protein) should therefore be based on the following:

Wineglassful of fruit juice such as apple or orange or pineapple.

Lightly cooked egg either poached, lightly boiled or scrambled (never fried) or cheese pudding or vegetarian savoury made from peas, beans, lentils and nuts (only one helping of protein to be taken at this meal).

Steamed or casseroled vegetables but NO POTATOES.

Dessert: Fresh acid fruit such as oranges, pears, grapes, grapefruit, any kind of berry.

This means that flesh food, fish, fried foods, milk puddings, heavy desserts, tea and coffee must not be taken at the midday meal. The reason for stopping potatoes is because it has been proved that a mixture of protein foods and starchy foods tends to bring about overeating and excessive weight.

Another week should elapse before the third meal is changed but even by this time some loss in weight will be felt; ideally this should be about one to two pounds a week. The third meal is the starchy one and is needed to give heat and energy. The person who is reducing must limit the starches and naturally she will feel the cold much more severely. This feeling will soon pass as the blood chemistry changes.

## THE THIRD MEAL

This should consist of a large raw salad using every kind

of vegetable in season. In addition any kind of fruit may be used with lemon juice as a dressing. For the rest of the meal, choose from wholewheat bread or scone or fruit cake, crisp bread, oatcakes, brown digestive biscuit. Only small quantities of the starchy foods are allowed—equal to about three small slices of wholewheat bread daily.

Butter and honey are permitted in small quantities.

SUPPER

This should consist of fresh acid fruit only such as apples, pears, oranges, grapes, grapefruit, lemons, plums and all forms of berries.

By this time the weight loss will be quite noticeable, but no attempt should be made to lose more than two pounds each week. A loss of this amount will not affect the blood pressure adversely. On this diet you will feel lighter and fresher in every way and should rise from the table hungry, a condition essential to health.

Gradually more exercise should be taken, and with the reduction in weight, this is a much easier matter. As previously mentioned, walking is the best exercise at this stage. If you are unaccustomed to walking very far, sharp inclines should be avoided at first. Later on, longer distances can be attempted and it will be found that even steep hills do not present the same difficulty. Movement is life to the over-stout and once the patient feels capable, a general scheme of exercises should be practised in the privacy of the home. These can be studied under *Exercises for Women* dealt with in the next chapter.

## Water Treatments

Water treatments are extremely helpful in reducing excessive weight and the morning quick cold bath and the cold compress at night will be most beneficial. Epsom salt baths, steam and Turkish baths can be taken occasionally.

It is essential that the treatment of weight reduction

should be from the viewpoint of health. Obesity is a disease, usually of mild form, but it is still a sign of potential ill-health and can be cured by helping the body to return to its normal state.

I would stress that three factors are required for health. A balanced diet which ensures that the body receives the food and vital mineral salts needed for correct functioning; sufficient physical activity and rest; and normal positive control of thoughts and emotions. If these three necessities are fulfilled the body will attain its normal weight, consistent with bone development and muscular formation.

# 16.
# Exercises for Women

WHEN A PATIENT is advised to practice some exercise it is common for her to remark that she gets enough exercise in performing her normal duties. This is only partially true because only certain muscles are used and very soon they become strong enough to perform the ordinary duties without overstrain. The other muscles, however, which are not used atrophy to some extent, and it is usually in these parts that ill-health begins, because the circulation is always deficient when the muscles are not used to the limit.

The following system of exercises is designed therefore to exercise all the vital parts of the body and if they are performed at least once a day, until there is a slight feeling of fatigue, they will prove of great aid in bringing health to the body.

Many women suffer from continual headache, eye

strain, poor hair and facial neuralgia, because they allow the neck to become tense, and the following simple exercise, performed at any time will bring about a great feeling of relaxation of the area.

## Neck Rolling

### *Exercise One*

Roll the head in as large a circle as possible to the right. Do this six times. Then roll to the left six times. During this exercise it is common to find that creakings and crackings are heard and felt. This need not cause alarm because it is only a sign that exercise is needed to relieve tenseness.

Sometimes this exercise will result in a slight giddiness and if this occurs, the following movement should be practised a few times to regain stability.

### *Exercise Two*

Bend the head straight forward until the chin touches the chest. Then bend it straight backward making an effort to touch the upper back with the back of the head. This movement equalizes the blood flow and allows the patient to regain her balance. Do not overstrain on the backward movement.

These two simple movements, practised at any odd time will do much to relieve tension in the neck and upper part of the body and will remove congestion from the head.

## Breathing

Anaemia and poor circulation are generally the result of deficient breathing and most women are very guilty of shallow chest movement. Real deep breathing should accompany physical exertion but this is not always possible, with the result that we have to practise deep breathing as an exercise.

*Exercise Three*

Stand erect with hands at the side. Breathe in and at the same time, lift the arms forward and upwards above the head. Hold the breath for a few seconds and then exhale slowly, lowering the arms to their original position. This is the most simple of all breathing exercises and yet it is sufficient to rejuvenate the entire body if practised night and morning for five minutes.

**Abdomen**

Many of our troubles originate in the abdominal region and special attention must be paid to keeping this part of the body in good muscular tone. Abdominal exercises are not easy to perform correctly and require a certain amount of perseverance. At the same time they are very valuable after childbirth and during the menopause when there is a definite tendency for the abdominal organs to sag.

*Exercise Four*

Stand erect with the hands clasped behind the back. Relax the abdomen as much as possible, then attempt to lift it slowly inward and then upward as high as possible. Once this position is obtained hold it for a few seconds before again relaxing. Continue to do this exercise until the muscles are slightly tired.

*Exercise Five*

Lie on back. Lift both legs straight upwards until they are at right angles with the floor. The legs must be kept perfectly straight. Lower slowly, still keeping the legs straight and without allowing the body to rise from the floor. Practise until slightly fatigued. If it is felt that this exercise is too severe then practise with one leg at a time until the muscles become stronger.

*Exercise Six*

Lie on back. Keeping the legs down and straight, lift the body forward and touch the toes. Do not allow the legs to rise. This is a powerful movement and may require considerable practice. At first the feet may be placed under a settee to give support to the action.

*Exercise Seven*

Lie on back, then raise the legs above the head and support them there with the hands on the hips. The weight of the legs and thighs should be taken on the shoulders. Try to retain this position as long as possible. This is an ideal exercise for anyone suffering from prolapse of the womb.

*Exercise Eight*

Retain the same position as the above exercise and practise:

1. 'Cycling'–throwing the legs as high as possible.
2. 'Scissors'–opening and crossing the legs.

**Inclined Board Exercises**

One of the most useful types of apparatus for exercising the lower abdomen and correcting many of the ailments of the reproductive system is the inclined board. This is a board about fifteen inches broad and some five feet long and fixed so that one end is supported about eighteen inches from the floor. This can easily be made by a carpenter and will soon repay the modest outlay. Two straps to catch the feet are connected to the higher end, and all exercises are done with the head nearest the floor.

**Anterior Displacements of the Womb**

Shown by irritation of the bladder at period time. Lie face upwards on the board and place the feet between the straps. Slowly raise the body upwards and reach as far as possible above the feet. Do this until slightly fatigued but do not overstrain because it is a very strenuous exercise. It is especially valuable just before and during the actual menstrual flow when the parts are suffused with blood.

**Posterior Displacement of the Womb**

Shown by irritation or constipation of the lower bowel. Lie face downwards on the inclined board and attempt to raise the body upwards by tensing the large muscles of the back. This is also a very strenuous exercise and must be done most carefully.

The inclined board may be used freely for all sorts of abdominal complaints, including obesity, prolapse, constipation and even digestive troubles. The value of the board is that the organs are always forced towards their natural position by the inclination.

It still must be stressed that a good walk each day is ideal for the circulation and should be taken whenever possible.